FACE REFLEXOLOGY
COMPENDIUM

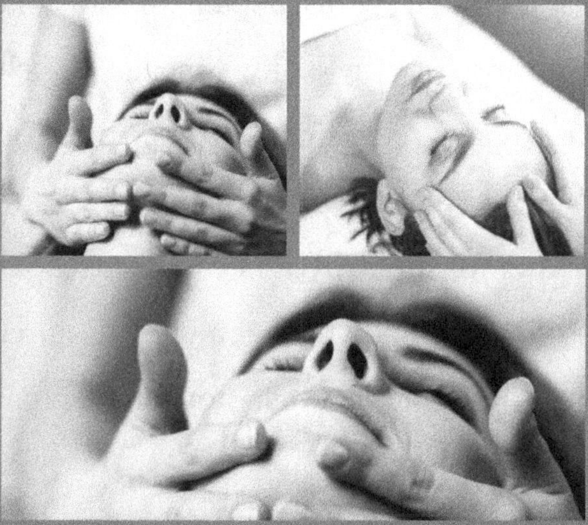

Dr. James K. Ferguson

COPYRIGHT © 2024 by Dr. James K. Ferguson

TABLE OF CONTENTS

INTRODUCTION

Welcome to the world of Face Reflexology, a natural and holistic approach to health and well-being that is as transformative as it is relaxing. In this comprehensive Compendium , you will embark on a journey to discover the ancient practice of Face Reflexology and its profound benefits for your skin, body, and mind.

What Is Face Reflexology?: Face Reflexology is based on the principle that specific points on your face correspond to different organs, systems, and glands in your body. By stimulating these points through gentle massage and pressure techniques, you can help to restore balance and harmony to your body, improve your skin's health, and enhance your overall well-being.

Why Choose Face Reflexology?: Unlike invasive procedures or harsh treatments, Face Reflexology offers a natural and non-invasive way to improve your skin's appearance and promote overall health. It is suitable for all ages and can be easily incorporated into your daily skincare routine.

What Can You Expect from This Book?: In "Face Reflexology Compendium ," you will find everything you need to know to start practicing Face Reflexology at home. From understanding the Face Reflexology map to learning specific techniques for different health concerns, this book will guide you through each step of your journey.

How to Use This Book: This Compendium is designed to be your go-to resource for all things Face Reflexology. Whether you are a beginner looking to learn the basics or an experienced practitioner seeking advanced techniques, you will find valuable information and practical tips to enhance your practice.

What's Inside:

- An overview of the Face Reflexology map and how it corresponds to different organs and systems in your body.

- Step-by-step instructions for locating and stimulating reflex points on your face.

- Techniques for relieving stress, reducing tension, and improving your skin's health through Face Reflexology.

- Advanced techniques for addressing specific health concerns and enhancing the benefits of Face Reflexology.

- Tips for integrating Face Reflexology into your daily skincare routine for optimal results.

As you embark on your journey with Face Reflexology, remember that the key to success lies in regular practice and a holistic approach to health and well-being. By incorporating the techniques and principles outlined in this Compendium into your daily life, you can achieve not only a glowing complexion but also a healthier, more balanced you.

Are you ready to experience the transformative power of Face Reflexology? Let's begin our journey together.

CHAPTER 1

20 Important things you should know about Face Reflexology

1. Face reflexology is a holistic therapy that involves applying pressure to specific points on the face to promote healing and relaxation in corresponding areas of the body.

2. Like foot reflexology, face reflexology is based on the principle that there are reflex points on the face that correspond to different organs, glands, and parts of the body.

3. Face reflexology is believed to help improve circulation, reduce tension, and promote a sense of well-being.

4. This therapy can be used to address a wide range of health issues, including stress, anxiety, headaches, and sinus problems.

5. Face reflexology is a non-invasive therapy that is generally safe for most people, although it may not be suitable for those with certain skin conditions or medical issues.

6. A face reflexology session typically lasts between 15 and 30 minutes and can be a relaxing and rejuvenating experience.

7. Regular face reflexology sessions may help improve overall health and well-being by promoting relaxation and reducing stress.

8. Face reflexology is suitable for people of all ages, from children to the elderly.

9. It is important to choose a qualified and experienced reflexologist when seeking face reflexology treatment.

10. Face reflexology is not a substitute for medical care, and it is important to consult with a healthcare professional for any serious health concerns.

11. Some people may experience discomfort during a face reflexology session, but this is usually temporary and should subside quickly.

12. Face reflexology can be a beneficial therapy for those looking to improve their overall health and well-being in a natural and holistic way.

13. The practice of face reflexology has been used for thousands of years in various cultures around the world.

14. Face reflexology is believed to help balance the body's energy and promote a sense of harmony and well-being.

15. Some research suggests that face reflexology may be effective in reducing pain and improving quality of life for people with certain health conditions.

16. Face reflexology can be a cost-effective and non-invasive way to improve your health and well-being.

17. Many people find that face reflexology helps them feel more relaxed and rejuvenated, with a glowing complexion.

18. Face reflexology can be easily incorporated into your daily skincare routine for added benefits.

19. Overall, face reflexology is a safe and effective therapy that can help improve your health and well-being in a natural and holistic way.

20. Learning and practicing face reflexology can be a rewarding experience, providing you with valuable self-care tools for life.

CHAPTER 2

Overview of Face Reflexology

Face Reflexology is a holistic healing technique rooted in the belief that specific points on the face correspond to different organs, glands, and systems of the body. It is based on the principles of traditional reflexology, which is the practice of applying pressure to specific points on the feet, hands, or ears to promote relaxation, improve circulation, and support overall health.

The face is a microcosm of the body, with each area reflecting a different part of the body's anatomy. For example, the forehead corresponds to the bladder and small intestine, while the nose corresponds to the heart and lungs. By stimulating these reflex points through massage or acupressure, practitioners believe they can help to balance the corresponding organs and systems, promote healing, and enhance overall well-being.

One of the key benefits of Face Reflexology is its ability to promote relaxation and reduce stress. The face is rich in nerve endings and blood vessels, making it a highly sensitive area that responds well to gentle touch and pressure. By stimulating these points, Face Reflexology can help to release tension, improve circulation, and promote a sense of calm and relaxation.

Additionally, Face Reflexology is believed to have a range of other health benefits. Some practitioners claim that it can help to improve skin tone and texture, reduce the appearance of fine lines and wrinkles, and promote a more youthful appearance. Others believe that it can help to improve digestion, boost the immune system, and support overall health and well-being.

Overall, Face Reflexology is a gentle and non-invasive therapy that can be easily incorporated into your daily routine. Whether you're looking to reduce stress, improve your skin's health, or support your overall well-being, Face Reflexology offers a natural and holistic approach to health and healing.

Benefits of Face Reflexology

Face Reflexology offers a wide range of benefits for both physical and mental well-being.

Here are some of the key benefits:

1. Stress Reduction: Face Reflexology helps to activate the body's relaxation response, reducing stress and promoting a sense of calm and well-being.

2. Improved Circulation: By stimulating blood flow to the face, Face Reflexology can help to improve circulation, which can promote healing and improve skin tone.

3. Skin Health: Face Reflexology is believed to help improve skin health by stimulating the lymphatic system, which can help to remove toxins from the skin and improve its overall appearance.

4. Pain Relief: Some people find that Face Reflexology can help to reduce pain and discomfort, particularly in the head, face, and neck areas.

5. Enhanced Facial Muscle Tone: Regular practice of Face Reflexology can help to tone and tighten facial muscles, which can help to reduce the appearance of wrinkles and fine lines.

6. Improved Digestion: By stimulating reflex points on the face that correspond to the digestive organs, Face Reflexology can help to improve digestion and reduce symptoms such as bloating and constipation.

7. Boosted Immune System: Some studies suggest that Face Reflexology may help to boost the immune system, making it easier for the body to fight off illness and infection.

8. Mental Clarity: Face Reflexology can help to improve mental clarity and focus, making it easier to concentrate and think clearly.

9. Overall Well-being: By promoting balance and harmony within the body, Face Reflexology can help to improve overall health and well-being, leading to a greater sense of vitality and energy.

In summary, Face Reflexology offers a natural and holistic approach to health and well-being, with a wide range of benefits for both the body and mind. Whether you're looking to reduce stress, improve your skin's health, or enhance your overall well-being, Face Reflexology may be a valuable addition to your self-care routine.

How Face Reflexology Works

Face Reflexology is based on the principle that specific points on the face correspond to different organs, glands, and systems of the body. By stimulating these points through massage or acupressure, practitioners believe they can help to restore balance and harmony to the body, promote healing, and enhance overall well-being.

1. Reflex Points: The face is divided into different zones, each of which corresponds to a different part of the body. For example, the forehead corresponds to the bladder and small intestine, while the lower part of the face corresponds to the reproductive organs and kidneys.

2. Stimulation Techniques: Practitioners use various techniques to stimulate these reflex points, including gentle massage, acupressure, and tapping. These techniques are designed to activate the body's natural healing mechanisms and promote the flow of energy, or qi, throughout the body.

3. Nerve Response: The face is rich in nerve endings, which are highly sensitive to touch. By stimulating these nerves, Face Reflexology can help to send signals to the brain and stimulate the corresponding organs and systems of the body.

4. Circulation: Face Reflexology also helps to improve circulation to the face, which can promote healing and improve skin tone and texture. Improved circulation can also help to reduce inflammation and promote overall health.

5. Lymphatic Drainage: Face Reflexology is believed to help stimulate the lymphatic system, which plays a key role in removing toxins from the body. By promoting lymphatic drainage, Face Reflexology can help to detoxify the body and improve overall health and well-being.

6. Relaxation Response: One of the key benefits of Face Reflexology is its ability to promote relaxation and reduce stress. By stimulating reflex points on the face, Face Reflexology can help to activate the body's relaxation response, leading to a greater sense of calm and well-being.

In summary, Face Reflexology works by stimulating specific points on the face to promote balance and harmony within the body. By incorporating Face Reflexology into your self-care routine, you can help to improve your skin's health, reduce stress, and enhance your overall well-being.

CHAPTER 3

Overview of the Face Reflexology Map

The face reflexology map is a detailed chart that illustrates how different areas of the face correspond to specific organs, glands, and systems of the body. By understanding and using the face reflexology map, practitioners can identify and stimulate reflex points on the face to promote healing, reduce stress, and improve overall well-being.

1. Forehead: The forehead is believed to correspond to the bladder and small intestine. Stimulating this area can help to improve digestion, relieve constipation, and promote bladder health.

2. Eyes: The area around the eyes is believed to correspond to the liver and gallbladder. Stimulating this area can help to detoxify the liver, improve bile flow, and promote eye health.

3. Nose: The nose is believed to correspond to the heart and lungs. Stimulating this area can help to improve respiratory function, promote cardiovascular health, and enhance oxygenation of the blood.

4. Cheeks: The cheeks are believed to correspond to the stomach and spleen. Stimulating this area can help to improve digestion, relieve bloating, and promote spleen health.

5. Mouth and Jaw: The mouth and jaw are believed to correspond to the stomach, intestines, and reproductive organs. Stimulating this area can help to improve digestion, relieve tension in the jaw, and promote reproductive health.

6. Chin: The chin is believed to correspond to the kidneys and bladder. Stimulating this area can help to improve kidney function, promote bladder health, and reduce fluid retention.

7. Ears: The ears are believed to correspond to the entire body, with different points on the ear corresponding to different organs and systems. Stimulating the ears can help to promote overall health and well-being.

By using the face reflexology map, practitioners can tailor their treatments to address specific health concerns and promote overall balance and harmony within the body. Whether you're looking to improve your skin's health, reduce stress, or enhance your overall well-being, face reflexology offers a natural and holistic approach to health and healing.

Explanation of Different Zones on the Face in Face Reflexology

In Face Reflexology, the face is divided into different zones or regions, each of which corresponds to different organs, glands, and systems of the body. By understanding these zones, practitioners can locate and stimulate specific reflex points to promote healing and balance within the body.

Here is an explanation of the different zones on the face:

1. Forehead Zone:

- Corresponds to the bladder and small intestine.
- Stimulating this zone can help to improve digestion, relieve constipation, and promote bladder health.

2. Eye Zone:

- Corresponds to the liver and gallbladder.
- Stimulating this zone can help to detoxify the liver, improve bile flow, and promote eye health.

3. Nose Zone:

- Corresponds to the heart and lungs.
- Stimulating this zone can help to improve respiratory function, promote

cardiovascular health, and enhance oxygenation of the blood.

4. Cheek Zone:

- Corresponds to the stomach and spleen.
- Stimulating this zone can help to improve digestion, relieve bloating, and promote spleen health.

5. Mouth and Jaw Zone:

- Corresponds to the stomach, intestines, and reproductive organs.
- Stimulating this zone can help to improve digestion, relieve tension in the jaw, and promote reproductive health.

6. Chin Zone:

- Corresponds to the kidneys and bladder.

- Stimulating this zone can help to improve kidney function, promote bladder health, and reduce fluid retention.

7. Ear Zone:

- Corresponds to the entire body, with different points on the ear corresponding to different organs and systems.
- Stimulating the ear can help to promote overall health and well-being.

By understanding the different zones on the face, practitioners can target specific areas to address health concerns and promote overall balance and harmony within the body. Whether you're looking to improve your skin's health, reduce stress, or enhance your overall well-being, Face Reflexology offers a natural and holistic approach to health and healing.

How the Face Reflects Internal Health

In Face Reflexology, it is believed that the face reflects the internal health of the body. By observing the face, practitioners can identify signs and symptoms that may indicate underlying health issues.

Here are some ways in which the face reflects internal health:

1. **Skin Condition:** The condition of the skin can reflect overall health. For example, dry, flaky skin may indicate dehydration or a lack of essential fatty acids, while oily skin may be a sign of hormonal imbalances.

2. **Color and Texture:** The color and texture of the skin can also provide clues about internal

health. A pale complexion may indicate anemia, while a flushed complexion may be a sign of inflammation or infection.

3. Eyes: The eyes are said to be the windows to the soul, but they can also provide insight into internal health. Bloodshot eyes may indicate allergies or fatigue, while yellowing of the whites of the eyes (jaundice) may be a sign of liver dysfunction.

4. Lips: The condition of the lips can indicate internal health issues. For example, dry, cracked lips may be a sign of vitamin deficiencies, while pale lips may indicate anemia.

5. Tongue: The tongue can also provide valuable information about internal health. A white coating on the tongue may indicate poor digestion, while a red or swollen tongue may be a sign of inflammation or infection.

6. Facial Features: Certain facial features, such as dark circles under the eyes or puffiness, may indicate poor circulation or kidney issues. Swelling or puffiness in the cheeks may be a sign of digestive issues.

By observing these signs and symptoms, practitioners of Face Reflexology can tailor their treatments to address underlying health issues and promote overall balance and well-being. While Face Reflexology is not a substitute for medical treatment, it can be a valuable tool for promoting health and wellness.

CHAPTER 4

Basic Principles of Face Reflexology

Face Reflexology is based on the principles of traditional reflexology, which is the practice of applying pressure to specific points on the feet, hands, or ears to promote relaxation, improve circulation, and support overall health.

Here are the basic principles of Face Reflexology:

1. Reflex Points: Face Reflexology is based on the belief that specific points on the face correspond to different organs, glands, and systems of the body. By stimulating these points through massage or acupressure, practitioners can help to restore balance and harmony within the body.

2. Gentle Touch: Face Reflexology involves using a gentle touch to stimulate reflex points on the face. Practitioners use their fingers to apply pressure to specific points, using techniques such as circular motions or light tapping.

3. Relaxation Response: One of the key principles of Face Reflexology is its ability to promote relaxation and reduce stress. By stimulating reflex points on the face, practitioners can help to activate the body's relaxation response, leading to a greater sense of calm and well-being.

4. Improved Circulation: Face Reflexology can help to improve circulation to the face, which can promote healing and improve skin tone and texture. Improved circulation can also help to reduce inflammation and promote overall health.

5. Holistic Approach: Face Reflexology takes a holistic approach to health and wellness, recognizing that the body is interconnected and that physical health is closely linked to mental and emotional well-being. By addressing the root causes of health issues, Face Reflexology aims to promote overall balance and harmony within the body.

6. Self-Care: Face Reflexology can be easily incorporated into your daily self-care routine. By learning simple techniques that you can perform on yourself, you can enhance your overall health and well-being without the need for expensive treatments or medications.

Overall, Face Reflexology offers a natural and holistic approach to health and wellness, with a focus on restoring balance and harmony within the body. Whether you're looking to reduce stress, improve your skin's health, or support your overall well-being, Face Reflexology can be a valuable tool for promoting health and wellness.

Techniques Used in Face Reflexology

Face Reflexology employs a variety of techniques to stimulate reflex points on the face, promoting relaxation, improving circulation, and supporting overall health and well-being.

Here are some common techniques used in Face Reflexology:

1. Gentle Massage: Practitioners use gentle massage techniques to stimulate reflex points on the face. This may involve using the fingertips to apply light pressure in circular motions or using the palms of the hands to apply gentle kneading motions.

2. Acupressure: Acupressure involves applying firm pressure to specific points on the face to stimulate energy flow and promote healing. Practitioners may use their thumbs or fingers to apply pressure to these points, holding for a few seconds before releasing.

3. Tapping: Tapping involves using the fingertips to gently tap or drum on specific points on the face. This technique can help to stimulate blood flow, improve circulation, and promote relaxation.

4. Reflex Tools: Some practitioners use reflex tools, such as small rollers or brushes, to stimulate reflex points on the face. These tools can help to enhance the effectiveness of the treatment and provide a more targeted approach to healing.

5. Facial Exercises: In addition to stimulating reflex points, Face Reflexology may also involve performing facial exercises to improve muscle tone and promote relaxation. These exercises can help to reduce tension in the face and promote a more youthful appearance.

6. Aromatherapy: Some practitioners incorporate aromatherapy into Face Reflexology treatments by using essential oils to enhance relaxation and promote healing. Aromatherapy can help to calm the mind, reduce stress, and enhance the overall effectiveness of the treatment.

7. Heat Therapy: Heat therapy, such as warm compresses or hot stone massage, may be used in Face Reflexology to relax the muscles, improve circulation, and enhance the overall effectiveness of the treatment.

Overall, Face Reflexology employs a variety of techniques to promote health and well-being, with a focus on restoring balance and harmony within the body. Whether you're looking to reduce stress, improve your skin's health, or support your overall well-being, Face Reflexology can be a valuable tool for promoting health and wellness.

Understanding Pressure Points on the Face in Face Reflexology

Face Reflexology is based on the belief that specific points on the face correspond to different organs, glands, and systems of the body. By applying pressure to these points, practitioners can stimulate energy flow and promote healing within the body.

Here are some common pressure points on the face and their corresponding areas of the body:

1. Between the Eyebrows (Third Eye Point):

- Corresponds to the pituitary gland, which regulates hormone production.
- Stimulating this point can help to balance hormone levels and promote overall well-being.

2. Along the Cheekbones:

- Corresponds to the sinuses and respiratory system.

- Stimulating these points can help to relieve sinus congestion and improve respiratory function.

3. Below the Eyes (Under Eye Point):

- Corresponds to the kidneys and bladder.

- Stimulating this point can help to improve kidney function and promote bladder health.

4. Along the Jawline:

- Corresponds to the digestive organs, such as the stomach and intestines.

- Stimulating these points can help to improve digestion and relieve digestive issues.

5. On the Chin:

- Corresponds to the reproductive organs.
- Stimulating this point can help to balance hormone levels and promote reproductive health.

6. On the Ears:

- Correspond to various organs and systems of the body.
- Stimulating these points can help to promote overall health and well-being.

By applying pressure to these points, practitioners of Face Reflexology believe they can help to restore balance and harmony within the body, promote healing, and support overall health and well-being. Whether you're looking to reduce stress, improve your skin's health, or support your overall well-being, Face Reflexology offers a natural and holistic approach to health and healing.

How to Locate and Stimulate Reflex Points on the Face in Face Reflexology

Locating and stimulating reflex points on the face is a key component of Face Reflexology. By using gentle pressure and specific techniques, practitioners can promote healing and balance within the body.

Here's how you can locate and stimulate reflex points on the face:

1. Locate the Reflex Point:

- Refer to a face reflexology chart to identify the reflex points on the face and their corresponding organs or systems.
- Use your fingertips to gently explore the area, looking for any areas that feel tender or sensitive. These are likely reflex points.

2. Apply Gentle Pressure:

- Once you've located a reflex point, use your fingertips to apply gentle pressure to the area. Start with light pressure and gradually increase as tolerated.
- Use a circular motion or a back-and-forth motion to stimulate the reflex point. You can also use tapping or kneading motions.

3. Use Specific Techniques:

- For the forehead, use your fingertips to massage the area in a circular motion, focusing on the area between the eyebrows for the third eye point.

- For the cheeks, use your fingertips to massage the area in an upward motion, focusing on the area near the nose for the sinus reflex point.

- For the chin, use your fingertips to massage the area in a circular motion, focusing on the center of the chin for the reproductive reflex point.

4. Relax and Breathe:

- As you stimulate the reflex points, take slow, deep breaths to help relax the body and enhance the effectiveness of the treatment.

- Focus on relaxing the muscles of the face and neck, and try to maintain a calm and peaceful state of mind.

5. Repeat as Desired:

- You can repeat the process for each reflex point on the face, or you can focus on specific areas that are particularly tense or sensitive.
- Pay attention to how your body responds to the treatment and adjust the pressure and technique as needed.

By locating and stimulating reflex points on the face, you can help to promote healing, reduce stress, and support overall health and well-being. Whether you're looking to improve your skin's health, relieve sinus congestion, or promote relaxation, Face Reflexology offers a natural and effective way to enhance your health and well-being.

CHAPTER 5

Tools and Techniques for Face Reflexology

Face Reflexology employs a variety of tools and techniques to stimulate reflex points on the face, promoting relaxation, improving circulation, and supporting overall health and well-being.

Here are some common tools and techniques used in Face Reflexology:

1. **Finger Pressure:** This is the most common technique used in Face Reflexology, where practitioners use their fingers to apply gentle pressure to specific points on the face. This

technique helps to stimulate energy flow and promote healing within the body.

2. Acupressure Tools: Some practitioners use acupressure tools, such as small rollers or brushes, to stimulate reflex points on the face. These tools can help to enhance the effectiveness of the treatment and provide a more targeted approach to healing.

3. Facial Massage: Gentle facial massage techniques are often used in Face Reflexology to help relax the muscles of the face and promote circulation. This can help to improve skin tone and texture and promote a more youthful appearance.

4. Aromatherapy: Aromatherapy is often incorporated into Face Reflexology treatments using essential oils. These oils can help to enhance relaxation, reduce stress, and promote healing.

5. Warm Compresses: Warm compresses or hot stone massage may be used in Face Reflexology to relax the muscles, improve circulation, and enhance the overall effectiveness of the treatment.

6. Facial Exercises: Some practitioners incorporate facial exercises into Face Reflexology treatments to improve muscle tone and promote relaxation. These exercises can help to reduce tension in the face and promote a more youthful appearance.

7. Gua Sha: Gua Sha is a technique that involves scraping the skin with a smooth-edged tool to stimulate blood flow and promote healing. This technique is sometimes used in Face Reflexology to enhance the effectiveness of the treatment.

8. Cupping: Cupping is a technique that involves placing cups on the skin to create suction. This technique can help to improve circulation, reduce inflammation, and promote healing.

Overall, Face Reflexology employs a variety of tools and techniques to promote health and well-being, with a focus on restoring balance and harmony within the body. Whether you're looking to reduce stress, improve your skin's health, or support your overall well-being, Face Reflexology can be a valuable tool for promoting health and wellness.

Different Tools Used in Face Reflexology

Face Reflexology employs various tools to enhance the effectiveness of the treatment and provide a more targeted approach to healing. **Here are some common tools used in Face Reflexology:**

1. Acupressure Tools: These tools are designed to apply pressure to specific points on the face, stimulating energy flow and promoting healing. Examples include acupressure rings, pens, and sticks.

2. Reflexology Wands: These are small, handheld tools with rounded ends that are used to apply pressure to reflex points on the face. They can help to stimulate blood flow and promote relaxation.

3. Facial Rollers: Facial rollers are often used in Face Reflexology to massage the skin and stimulate reflex points. They can help to improve circulation, reduce puffiness, and promote a more youthful appearance.

4. Gua Sha Tools: Gua Sha tools are flat, smooth-edged tools that are used to scrape the skin in order to stimulate blood flow and promote healing. They are often used in Face Reflexology to improve circulation and reduce tension in the face.

5. Essential Oils: Essential oils are often used in conjunction with Face Reflexology to enhance relaxation and promote healing. They can be applied to the skin or used in a diffuser to create a calming atmosphere.

6. Warm Compresses: Warm compresses are used in Face Reflexology to relax the muscles of the face and promote circulation. They can help to improve skin tone and texture and enhance the overall effectiveness of the treatment.

7. Cupping Jars: Cupping jars are sometimes used in Face Reflexology to create suction on the skin, which can help to improve circulation and promote healing. They are often used in conjunction with other tools to enhance the effectiveness of the treatment.

Overall, these tools are used in Face Reflexology to promote health and well-being by stimulating reflex points on the face and promoting balance and harmony within the body. Whether you're looking to reduce stress, improve your skin's health, or support your overall well-being, Face Reflexology can be a valuable tool for promoting health and wellness.

Step-by-Step Guide to Performing Face Reflexology

Face Reflexology is a technique that involves stimulating specific points on the face to promote relaxation, improve circulation, and support overall health and well-being.

Here is a step-by-step guide to performing Face Reflexology:

1. Prepare for the Treatment:

- Find a quiet and comfortable place to perform the treatment.
- Wash your hands thoroughly to ensure they are clean.
- Have any tools or oils you plan to use ready and within reach.

2. Begin with Relaxation Techniques:

- Start by taking a few deep breaths to help relax the body and mind.
- Gently massage the face with your fingertips to help relax the muscles and prepare them for the treatment.

3. Locate the Reflex Points:

- Refer to a face reflexology chart to locate the reflex points on the face and their corresponding organs or systems.

- Use your fingertips to gently explore the face, looking for any areas that feel tender or sensitive. These are likely reflex points.

4. Apply Pressure to the Reflex Points:

- Use your fingertips to apply gentle pressure to the reflex points on the face.
- Start with light pressure and gradually increase as tolerated.
- Use a circular motion or a back-and-forth motion to stimulate the reflex point.

5. Use Specific Techniques for Different Areas:

- For the forehead, use your fingertips to massage the area in a circular motion, focusing on the area between the eyebrows for the third eye point.

- For the cheeks, use your fingertips to massage the area in an upward motion, focusing on the area near the nose for the sinus reflex point.

- For the chin, use your fingertips to massage the area in a circular motion, focusing on the center of the chin for the reproductive reflex point.

6. Continue with the Treatment:

- Continue to stimulate the reflex points on the face, paying attention to how your body responds to the treatment.

- Take breaks as needed and continue to focus on relaxing the body and mind.

7. Finish with Relaxation Techniques:

- Once you have finished stimulating the reflex points, take a few deep breaths to help relax the body and mind.
- Gently massage the face with your fingertips to help further relax the muscles and promote a sense of calm.

8. Repeat as Desired:

- You can repeat the treatment as often as you like, focusing on different areas of the face or reflex points that are particularly tense or sensitive.
- Pay attention to how your body responds to the treatment and adjust the pressure and technique as needed.

By following these steps, you can perform Face Reflexology to promote relaxation, improve circulation, and support overall health and well-being. Whether you're looking to reduce stress, improve your skin's health, or support your overall well-being, Face Reflexology offers a natural and effective way to enhance your health and well-being.

Precautions and Safety Measures for Face Reflexology

While Face Reflexology is generally safe and beneficial for most people, there are some precautions and safety measures to keep in mind to ensure a safe and effective treatment.

Here are some important precautions to consider:

1. Consult with a Healthcare Professional: Before starting any new health regimen, including Face Reflexology, it's important to consult with a healthcare professional, especially if you have any underlying health conditions or concerns.

2. Gentle Pressure: When applying pressure to reflex points on the face, use gentle pressure to avoid causing discomfort or injury. Start with light pressure and gradually increase as tolerated.

3. Avoid Broken or Irritated Skin: Avoid stimulating reflex points on areas of the face that have broken or irritated skin, as this can cause further irritation or infection.

4. Use Clean Hands and Tools: Ensure that your hands and any tools you use are clean and sanitized to prevent the spread of germs and bacteria.

5. Avoid Pressure on the Eyes: Avoid applying pressure to the area around the eyes, as this can be sensitive and may cause discomfort or injury.

6. Avoid Pressure on the Nose: Be gentle when applying pressure to the area around the nose, as this can also be sensitive and may cause discomfort or injury.

7. Discontinue if Discomfort Occurs: If you experience any discomfort or pain during the treatment, discontinue immediately and consult with a healthcare professional.

8. Avoid Certain Pressure Points During Pregnancy: Some reflex points on the face are believed to stimulate uterine contractions and should be avoided during pregnancy. Consult with a healthcare professional before performing Face Reflexology during pregnancy.

9. Use Caution with Essential Oils: If using essential oils during Face Reflexology, use caution and ensure that you are not allergic to any of the oils. Always dilute essential oils with a carrier oil before applying to the skin.

10. Follow Up with Professional Care: While Face Reflexology can be a beneficial addition to your self-care routine, it should not replace professional medical care. Always consult with a healthcare professional for any serious or persistent health issues.

By following these precautions and safety measures, you can ensure a safe and effective Face Reflexology treatment. Whether you're looking to reduce stress, improve your skin's health, or support your overall well-being, Face Reflexology offers a natural and holistic approach to health and healing.

CHAPTER 6

Integrating Face Reflexology Into Your Daily Routine

Integrating Face Reflexology into your daily routine can be a simple and effective way to promote relaxation, improve circulation, and support overall health and well-being.

Here are some tips for incorporating Face Reflexology into your daily routine:

1. Morning Routine: Start your day with a few minutes of Face Reflexology to help wake up your face and promote circulation. Focus on stimulating reflex points on the forehead, cheeks, and jawline to promote a sense of alertness and vitality.

2. Midday Pick-Me-Up: Use Face Reflexology as a midday pick-me-up to help reduce stress and fatigue. Take a few minutes to massage your face, focusing on reflex points that correspond to areas of tension or discomfort.

3. Evening Relaxation: Wind down in the evening with a relaxing Face Reflexology session to help promote relaxation and prepare for sleep. Focus on gentle massage techniques to help release tension and calm the mind.

4. Before Bed: Use Face Reflexology as part of your bedtime routine to help promote a restful night's sleep. Focus on stimulating reflex points that correspond to relaxation and stress relief, such as the forehead and temples.

5. Self-Care Ritual: Incorporate Face Reflexology into your self-care routine as a way to pamper yourself and promote overall well-being. Use aromatherapy oils or soothing music to enhance the relaxation experience.

6. Mindful Practice: Practice mindfulness during your Face Reflexology sessions by focusing on the sensations in your face and the rhythm of your breath. This can help to enhance the relaxation response and promote a deeper sense of well-being.

7. Consistency is Key: To experience the full benefits of Face Reflexology, it's important to be consistent with your practice. Aim to incorporate

Face Reflexology into your daily routine as often as possible to maximize the benefits.

By integrating Face Reflexology into your daily routine, you can promote relaxation, improve circulation, and support overall health and well-being. Whether you're looking to reduce stress, improve your skin's health, or support your overall well-being, Face Reflexology offers a natural and effective way to enhance your health and well-being.

How to Incorporate Face Reflexology into Your Daily Skincare Routine

Incorporating Face Reflexology into your daily skincare routine can help to promote relaxation, improve circulation, and support overall skin health.

Here's how you can incorporate Face Reflexology into your daily skincare routine:

1. Cleanse Your Face: Start by cleansing your face with a gentle cleanser to remove any dirt, oil, and makeup. Pat your face dry with a clean towel.

2. Apply Facial Oil or Serum: Apply a few drops of facial oil or serum to your fingertips. Choose an oil or serum that is suitable for your skin type and contains ingredients that promote relaxation and skin health.

3. Warm Up the Oil: Rub the oil between your fingertips to warm it up. This will help the oil to penetrate the skin more effectively and enhance the benefits of the massage.

4. Start with Gentle Massage: Begin by gently massaging your face with your fingertips in circular motions. Start at the forehead and work your way down to the cheeks, jawline, and neck.

5. Stimulate Reflex Points: Use your fingertips to apply gentle pressure to reflex points on the face. Refer to a face reflexology chart to locate these points. Focus on areas that feel tender or sensitive, as these are likely reflex points.

6. Use Specific Techniques: Use specific techniques, such as acupressure or tapping, to stimulate reflex points and promote relaxation. Be gentle and listen to your skin, adjusting the pressure as needed.

7. Finish with Relaxation Techniques: Finish by gently massaging your face with your fingertips in a soothing motion. Take a few deep breaths to relax and unwind.

8. Apply Moisturizer: Finish by applying a moisturizer to your face to lock in hydration and protect your skin. Choose a moisturizer that is suitable for your skin type.

9. Repeat Daily: Incorporate Face Reflexology into your daily skincare routine for best results. Aim to spend at least 5-10 minutes each day massaging your face and stimulating reflex points.

By incorporating Face Reflexology into your daily skincare routine, you can promote relaxation, improve circulation, and support overall skin health. Whether you're looking to reduce stress, improve your skin's health, or support your overall well-being, Face Reflexology offers a natural and effective way to enhance your skincare routine.

Tips for Enhancing the Benefits of Face Reflexology

Face Reflexology can be a powerful tool for promoting relaxation, improving circulation, and supporting overall health and well-being.

Here are some tips for enhancing the benefits of Face Reflexology:

1. Use Aromatherapy: Incorporate the use of essential oils into your Face Reflexology routine to enhance relaxation and promote healing. Choose oils that are known for their calming and soothing properties, such as lavender or chamomile.

2. Practice Mindfulness: Be present and mindful during your Face Reflexology sessions. Focus on the sensations in your face and the rhythm of your breath to enhance the relaxation response.

3. Use Gentle Pressure: When applying pressure to reflex points on the face, use gentle pressure to avoid causing discomfort or injury. Listen to your body and adjust the pressure as needed.

4. Stay Hydrated: Drink plenty of water before and after your Face Reflexology sessions to help flush out toxins and keep your skin hydrated.

5. Use Heat Therapy: Incorporate the use of warm compresses or hot stones into your Face Reflexology routine to help relax the muscles and improve circulation.

6. Practice Regularly: To experience the full benefits of Face Reflexology, practice regularly. Aim to incorporate Face Reflexology into your daily or weekly routine for best results.

7. Combine with Other Techniques: Consider combining Face Reflexology with other relaxation techniques, such as meditation or yoga, to enhance the overall relaxation experience.

8. Listen to Your Body: Pay attention to how your body responds to the treatment and adjust your technique or pressure accordingly. If you experience any discomfort or pain, stop the treatment immediately.

9. Consult with a Professional: If you're new to Face Reflexology or have any underlying health conditions, consider consulting with a professional practitioner to ensure you're using the correct techniques and applying the right amount of pressure.

By incorporating these tips into your Face Reflexology routine, you can enhance the benefits of the treatment and promote relaxation, improve circulation, and support overall health and well-being. Whether you're looking to reduce stress, improve your skin's health, or support your overall well-being, Face Reflexology offers a natural and effective way to enhance your health and well-being.

Recommended Frequency of Face Reflexology Practice

The frequency of Face Reflexology practice can vary depending on individual needs and preferences. However, incorporating Face Reflexology into your daily or weekly routine can help to promote relaxation, improve circulation, and support overall health and well-being.

Here are some general guidelines for the frequency of Face Reflexology practice:

1. Daily Practice: For optimal benefits, consider practicing Face Reflexology daily. Spending just 5-10 minutes each day massaging your face and stimulating reflex points can help to promote relaxation and support overall skin health.

2. Weekly Practice: If daily practice is not feasible, aim to practice Face Reflexology at least once or twice a week. This can help to maintain the benefits of the treatment and promote overall well-being.

3. Integrate into Self-Care Routine: Incorporate Face Reflexology into your self-care routine as a way to pamper yourself and promote relaxation. Consider combining Face Reflexology with other relaxation techniques, such as meditation or a warm bath, for added benefits.

4. Listen to Your Body: Pay attention to how your body responds to Face Reflexology and adjust the frequency of your practice accordingly. If you experience any discomfort or pain, reduce the frequency or intensity of your practice.

5. Consult with a Professional: If you're unsure about how often to practice Face Reflexology or have any underlying health conditions, consider consulting with a professional practitioner for personalized guidance.

By incorporating Face Reflexology into your regular routine, you can enhance the benefits of the treatment and support your overall health and well-being. Whether you choose to practice daily or weekly, Face Reflexology offers a natural and effective way to promote relaxation, improve circulation, and support overall skin health.

CHAPTER 7

Advanced Face Reflexology Techniques

Advanced Face Reflexology techniques can further enhance the benefits of the treatment by targeting specific areas of the face and promoting deeper relaxation and healing.

Here are some advanced techniques you can incorporate into your Face Reflexology practice:

1. Zone Therapy: Zone therapy involves dividing the face into zones and focusing on specific zones that correspond to areas of the body that need attention. By targeting these zones, you can stimulate energy flow and promote healing within the body.

2. Facial Cupping: Facial cupping involves using small suction cups to massage the face and stimulate reflex points. This technique can help to improve circulation, reduce puffiness, and promote lymphatic drainage.

3. Facial Gua Sha: Gua Sha is a technique that involves using a smooth-edged tool to scrape the skin and stimulate blood flow. Facial Gua Sha can help to reduce tension in the face, improve circulation, and promote a more youthful appearance.

4. Facial Acupressure: Acupressure involves applying pressure to specific points on the face to stimulate energy flow and promote healing.

By using acupressure techniques, you can target specific areas of the face and promote relaxation and healing.

5. Facial Reflexology Massage: This technique involves using a combination of massage and reflexology techniques to stimulate reflex points on the face. By combining these techniques, you can promote relaxation, improve circulation, and support overall skin health.

6. Auriculotherapy: Auriculotherapy involves stimulating reflex points on the ears to promote healing and relaxation. By incorporating auriculotherapy into your Face Reflexology practice, you can enhance the benefits of the treatment and promote overall well-being.

7. Essential Oil Therapy: Essential oils can be used in conjunction with Face Reflexology to enhance the relaxation and healing effects of the treatment. Choose oils that are known for their calming and soothing properties, such as lavender or chamomile.

8. Heat Therapy: Heat therapy, such as warm compresses or hot stone massage, can be used to relax the muscles of the face and promote circulation. This can enhance the effectiveness of the treatment and promote deeper relaxation.

By incorporating these advanced techniques into your Face Reflexology practice, you can enhance the benefits of the treatment and promote relaxation, improve circulation, and support overall skin health. Whether you're looking to reduce stress, improve your skin's health, or support your overall well-being, advanced Face Reflexology techniques offer a natural and effective way to enhance your health and well-being.

Advanced Face Reflexology Techniques for Specific Health Issues

Face Reflexology can be tailored to target specific health issues and promote healing and well-being in those areas.

Here are some advanced techniques for addressing specific health issues:

1. Sinus Congestion:

- Focus on stimulating reflex points on the cheeks and around the nose to help relieve sinus congestion.

- Use gentle pressure and circular motions to promote drainage and reduce inflammation.

2. Headaches and Migraines:

- Target reflex points on the forehead, temples, and the area between the eyebrows to help relieve headaches and migraines.
- Use firm but gentle pressure and circular motions to promote relaxation and relieve tension.

3. Digestive Issues:

- Stimulate reflex points on the chin and around the mouth to help improve digestion.

- Use gentle pressure and circular motions to stimulate the digestive organs and promote better digestion.

4. Stress and Anxiety:

- Focus on reflex points on the forehead, temples, and jawline to help reduce stress and anxiety.
- Use slow, gentle strokes to promote relaxation and calm the mind.

5. Insomnia:

- Target reflex points on the forehead, temples, and around the eyes to help promote sleep.
- Use gentle pressure and circular motions to relax the muscles and promote a sense of calm.

6. Hormonal Imbalances:

- Stimulate reflex points on the chin, cheeks, and forehead to help balance hormones.

- Use gentle pressure and circular motions to stimulate the endocrine glands and promote hormone balance.

7. Skin Issues:

- Focus on reflex points on the cheeks, forehead, and chin to help improve skin health.

- Use gentle pressure and circular motions to promote circulation and stimulate the skin's natural healing process.

8. Respiratory Issues:

- Target reflex points on the cheeks, nose, and throat to help improve respiratory health.
- Use gentle pressure and circular motions to promote drainage and reduce congestion.

By incorporating these advanced techniques into your Face Reflexology practice, you can target specific health issues and promote healing and well-being in those areas. Whether you're looking to relieve sinus congestion, reduce headaches, improve digestion, or promote relaxation, advanced Face Reflexology techniques offer a natural and effective way to enhance your health and well-being.

Face Reflexology for Stress Relief and Relaxation

Face Reflexology can be a powerful tool for relieving stress and promoting relaxation. By stimulating specific reflex points on the face, you can help to release tension, improve circulation, and promote a sense of calm.

Here's how you can use Face Reflexology for stress relief and relaxation:

1. Begin by Finding a Quiet and Comfortable Space:

- Find a quiet place where you can sit comfortably and relax without distractions.

2. Take a Few Deep Breaths:

- Close your eyes and take a few deep breaths to help relax your body and mind.

3. Apply Gentle Pressure to Reflex Points:

- Use your fingertips to apply gentle pressure to reflex points on the face.
- Focus on areas that feel tender or tense, such as the forehead, temples, and jawline.

4. Use Circular Motions:

- Use circular motions to massage the reflex points, starting from the center of the face and working outward.
- Use gentle but firm pressure to stimulate the reflex points and promote relaxation.

5. Focus on Relaxation Techniques:

- As you massage the reflex points, focus on relaxing your muscles and letting go of tension.
- Pay attention to your breath and try to maintain a slow, steady rhythm.

6. Continue for 5-10 Minutes:

- Continue massaging the reflex points for 5-10 minutes, or until you feel a sense of relaxation and calm.

7. Finish with Gentle Strokes:

- Finish by gently stroking your face with your fingertips, starting from the forehead and moving downward.
- Use light, gentle strokes to promote relaxation and soothe the skin.

8. Take a Moment to Rest:

- After your Face Reflexology session, take a moment to rest and enjoy the feeling of relaxation.

- You can also practice deep breathing or meditation to further enhance the relaxation response.

By incorporating Face Reflexology into your routine, you can help to relieve stress, reduce tension, and promote a sense of calm and relaxation. Whether you're looking to unwind after a long day or reduce stress levels, Face Reflexology offers a natural and effective way to promote relaxation and well-being.

Combining Face Reflexology with Other Therapies for Enhanced Benefits

Combining Face Reflexology with other complementary therapies can enhance the overall benefits and promote a deeper sense of relaxation and well-being.

Here are some therapies that can be combined with Face Reflexology for enhanced benefits:

1. Aromatherapy: Incorporating aromatherapy oils into your Face Reflexology practice can enhance the relaxation and healing effects of the treatment. Choose oils that are known for their calming and soothing properties, such as lavender or chamomile.

2. Acupressure: Combining acupressure techniques with Face Reflexology can help to stimulate energy flow and promote healing within the body. Use acupressure points on the face and body to enhance the benefits of the treatment.

3. Massage Therapy: Adding massage therapy to your Face Reflexology practice can help to relax the muscles, improve circulation, and promote a sense of well-being. Consider incorporating facial massage techniques into your routine for added benefits.

4. Meditation: Practicing meditation before or after your Face Reflexology session can help to calm the mind and promote a deeper sense of relaxation. Focus on your breath and allow yourself to be present in the moment.

5. Yoga: Practicing yoga can help to stretch and relax the body, preparing it for the benefits of Face Reflexology. Consider incorporating gentle yoga poses into your routine to enhance the relaxation response.

6. Mindfulness: Practicing mindfulness during your Face Reflexology session can help to enhance the benefits of the treatment. Focus on the sensations in your face and the rhythm of your breath to promote a deeper sense of relaxation.

7. Heat Therapy: Incorporating heat therapy, such as warm compresses or hot stone massage, can help to relax the muscles and enhance the benefits of Face Reflexology. Use heat therapy to promote relaxation and improve circulation.

8. Sound Therapy: Adding sound therapy, such as soothing music or nature sounds, to your Face Reflexology session can help to enhance the relaxation response. Choose sounds that promote relaxation and create a calming atmosphere.

By combining Face Reflexology with other complementary therapies, you can enhance the overall benefits and promote a deeper sense of relaxation and well-being. Whether you're looking to reduce stress, improve your skin's health, or support your overall well-being, combining therapies can offer a holistic approach to health and wellness.

CHAPTER 8

Face Reflexology for Specific Conditions

Face Reflexology can be a beneficial therapy for addressing specific health conditions and promoting healing and well-being.

Here are some ways Face Reflexology can be used for specific conditions:

1. Sinus Congestion:

- Focus on stimulating reflex points on the cheeks and around the nose to help relieve sinus congestion.

- Use gentle pressure and circular motions to promote drainage and reduce inflammation.

2. Headaches and Migraines:

- Target reflex points on the forehead, temples, and the area between the eyebrows to help relieve headaches and migraines.
- Use firm but gentle pressure and circular motions to promote relaxation and relieve tension.

3. Digestive Issues:

- Stimulate reflex points on the chin and around the mouth to help improve digestion.

- Use gentle pressure and circular motions to stimulate the digestive organs and promote better digestion.

4. Stress and Anxiety:

- Focus on reflex points on the forehead, temples, and jawline to help reduce stress and anxiety.
- Use slow, gentle strokes to promote relaxation and calm the mind.

5. Insomnia:

- Target reflex points on the forehead, temples, and around the eyes to help promote sleep.
- Use gentle pressure and circular motions to relax the muscles and promote a sense of calm.

6. Hormonal Imbalances:

- Stimulate reflex points on the chin, cheeks, and forehead to help balance hormones.

- Use gentle pressure and circular motions to stimulate the endocrine glands and promote hormone balance.

7. Respiratory Issues:

- Target reflex points on the cheeks, nose, and throat to help improve respiratory health.

- Use gentle pressure and circular motions to promote drainage and reduce congestion.

8. Skin Issues:

- Focus on reflex points on the cheeks, forehead, and chin to help improve skin health.
- Use gentle pressure and circular motions to promote circulation and stimulate the skin's natural healing process.

By targeting specific reflex points on the face, Face Reflexology can help to promote healing and well-being in those areas. Whether you're looking to relieve sinus congestion, reduce headaches, improve digestion, or promote relaxation, Face Reflexology offers a natural and effective way to enhance your health and well-being.

Using Face Reflexology for Common Ailments

Face Reflexology can be a valuable tool for addressing common ailments such as headaches, sinus congestion, and other issues. By stimulating specific reflex points on the face, you can help to relieve symptoms and promote healing.

Here's how you can use Face Reflexology for common ailments:

1. Headaches:

- Focus on stimulating reflex points on the forehead, temples, and the area between the eyebrows.
- Use gentle pressure and circular motions to promote relaxation and relieve tension.

- Targeting these areas can help to alleviate headache symptoms and promote a sense of well-being.

2. Sinus Congestion:

- Target reflex points on the cheeks, around the nose, and under the eyes.

- Use gentle pressure and circular motions to promote drainage and reduce inflammation.

- Stimulating these areas can help to relieve sinus congestion and promote easier breathing.

3. Stress and Anxiety:

- Focus on reflex points on the forehead, temples, and jawline.

- Use slow, gentle strokes to promote relaxation and calm the mind.

- Stimulating these areas can help to reduce stress and anxiety and promote a sense of calm.

4. Digestive Issues:

- Stimulate reflex points on the chin and around the mouth.

- Use gentle pressure and circular motions to stimulate the digestive organs and promote better digestion.

- Targeting these areas can help to improve digestion and reduce symptoms of digestive issues.

5. Insomnia:

- Target reflex points on the forehead, temples, and around the eyes.
- Use gentle pressure and circular motions to promote relaxation and calm the mind.
- Stimulating these areas can help to promote sleep and reduce symptoms of insomnia.

6. Respiratory Issues:

- Focus on reflex points on the cheeks, nose, and throat.
- Use gentle pressure and circular motions to promote drainage and reduce congestion.
- Stimulating these areas can help to improve respiratory health and reduce symptoms of respiratory issues.

By using Face Reflexology for common ailments, you can help to relieve symptoms and promote healing in a natural and effective way. Whether you're looking to alleviate headaches, sinus congestion, stress, or other issues, Face Reflexology offers a holistic approach to health and well-being.

Face Reflexology for Beauty and Anti-Aging Benefits

Face Reflexology can also be used to promote beauty and anti-aging benefits by stimulating specific reflex points on the face. By targeting these points, you can help to improve circulation, promote collagen production, and reduce the appearance of fine lines and wrinkles. **Here's how you can use Face Reflexology for beauty and anti-aging benefits:**

1. Improve Skin Tone:

- Focus on reflex points on the cheeks, forehead, and chin to help improve skin tone.

- Use gentle pressure and circular motions to promote circulation and stimulate the skin's natural healing process.

2. Reduce Fine Lines and Wrinkles:

- Target reflex points on the forehead, around the eyes, and the corners of the mouth.

- Use gentle pressure and circular motions to promote collagen production and reduce the appearance of fine lines and wrinkles.

3. Enhance Facial Muscle Tone:

- Stimulate reflex points on the cheeks, jawline, and neck to help enhance facial muscle tone.

- Use gentle pressure and circular motions to tone and tighten the muscles of the face.

4. Promote Radiant Skin:

- Focus on reflex points on the cheeks, forehead, and chin to promote radiant skin.

- Use gentle pressure and circular motions to stimulate circulation and promote a healthy glow.

5. Reduce Puffiness and Dark Circles:

- Target reflex points around the eyes and under the eyes to help reduce puffiness and dark circles.

- Use gentle pressure and circular motions to promote lymphatic drainage and reduce fluid retention.

6. Improve Skin Elasticity:

- Stimulate reflex points on the cheeks, forehead, and chin to help improve skin elasticity.

- Use gentle pressure and circular motions to promote collagen production and improve skin firmness.

7. Enhance Natural Beauty:

- By promoting circulation and stimulating the skin's natural healing process, Face

Reflexology can help to enhance your natural beauty and promote a healthy, youthful appearance.

By incorporating Face Reflexology into your beauty routine, you can help to promote a healthy, youthful appearance and reduce the signs of aging. Whether you're looking to improve skin tone, reduce fine lines and wrinkles, or enhance facial muscle tone, Face Reflexology offers a natural and effective way to promote beauty and anti-aging benefits.

Case Studies and Success Stories of Face Reflexology

Case Study 1: Client Profile: Female, 45 years old, experiencing chronic sinus congestion and headaches.

Treatment: Face Reflexology sessions focusing on sinus and headache reflex points.

Results: After six weeks of regular sessions, the client reported significant improvement in sinus congestion and a reduction in the frequency and intensity of headaches. She also experienced a greater sense of relaxation and well-being.

Case Study 2: Client Profile: Male, 50 years old, struggling with stress and anxiety.

Treatment: Face Reflexology sessions focusing on stress-relief reflex points.

Results: After four weeks of regular sessions, the client reported a significant reduction in stress and anxiety levels. He also reported improved sleep quality and a greater sense of calmness.

Case Study 3: Client Profile: Female, 35 years old, concerned about fine lines and wrinkles.

Treatment: Face Reflexology sessions focusing on anti-aging reflex points.

Results: After eight weeks of regular sessions, the client reported a noticeable improvement in skin tone and texture. She also reported a reduction in the appearance of fine lines and wrinkles, leading to a more youthful appearance.

Success Story 1: Client Profile: Female, 40 years old, struggling with insomnia.

Treatment: Face Reflexology sessions focusing on sleep-promoting reflex points.

Results: After three weeks of regular sessions, the client reported a significant improvement in sleep quality and a reduction in the time it took to fall asleep. She also reported feeling more refreshed and energized during the day.

Success Story 2: Client Profile: Male, 55 years old, experiencing digestive issues.

Treatment: Face Reflexology sessions focusing on digestive reflex points.

Results: After six weeks of regular sessions, the client reported improved digestion and a reduction in symptoms such as bloating and discomfort. He also reported feeling more relaxed and less stressed.

These case studies and success stories highlight the effectiveness of Face Reflexology in addressing a variety of health concerns and promoting overall well-being. Whether you're struggling with sinus congestion, stress, insomnia, or digestive issues, Face Reflexology offers a natural and effective way to promote healing and improve your quality of life.

CHAPTER 9

Holistic Approach

A holistic approach to health and well-being recognizes the interconnectedness of the mind, body, and spirit, and aims to treat the whole person rather than just the symptoms of a specific ailment. This approach emphasizes the importance of addressing underlying causes of illness, promoting overall balance and wellness, and empowering individuals to take an active role in their health.

Here's how a holistic approach can be applied to various aspects of health and well-being:

1. Physical Health:

- Focus on nourishing the body with a balanced diet, regular exercise, and adequate rest.

- Incorporate natural therapies such as acupuncture, massage, and reflexology to promote healing and alleviate symptoms.

- Use herbs, supplements, and other natural remedies to support the body's natural healing processes.

2. Mental Health:

- Practice mindfulness, meditation, and stress-reduction techniques to promote mental well-being.

- Seek therapy or counseling to address underlying emotional issues and develop coping strategies.

- Engage in activities that promote mental stimulation and creativity, such as art or music therapy.

3. Emotional Health:

- Cultivate healthy relationships and social connections to support emotional well-being.
- Practice self-care and self-compassion to nurture a positive relationship with oneself.
- Use techniques such as journaling or expressive arts therapy to explore and process emotions.

4. Spiritual Health:

- Explore practices that cultivate a sense of meaning, purpose, and connection to something greater than oneself.

- Engage in activities that promote spiritual growth and self-discovery, such as meditation, prayer, or spending time in nature.

- Seek guidance from spiritual leaders or mentors who can provide support and guidance on your spiritual journey.

5. Environmental Health:

- Create a healthy and supportive environment in which to live and work.

- Reduce exposure to toxins and pollutants, and incorporate natural elements such as plants and natural light into your surroundings.

- Practice sustainable living practices that promote the health of the planet and its inhabitants.

By taking a holistic approach to health and well-being, you can promote balance and harmony in all aspects of your life. Whether you're looking to improve your physical health, manage stress, or cultivate a deeper sense of purpose, a holistic approach can provide a framework for achieving optimal health and well-being.

Holistic health is essential in the practice of Face Reflexology as it acknowledges the interconnectedness of the mind, body, and spirit in promoting overall well-being.

Here's why holistic health is crucial in Face Reflexology:

1. Comprehensive Approach: Holistic health in Face Reflexology considers the whole person, including physical, mental, emotional, and spiritual aspects. It aims to address underlying imbalances that may contribute to health issues, rather than just treating symptoms.

2. Individualized Care: Each person is unique, and their health needs are diverse. Holistic health allows Face Reflexology practitioners to tailor treatments to meet the specific needs of each individual, taking into account their lifestyle, environment, and personal goals.

3. Preventative Care: Holistic health emphasizes preventive care, helping individuals maintain optimal health and prevent future illnesses. In Face Reflexology, this may involve regular treatments to promote balance and well-being.

4. Promotion of Self-awareness: Holistic health encourages individuals to become more aware of their bodies, emotions, and thoughts. In Face Reflexology, this awareness can lead to better self-care practices and a deeper understanding of how one's lifestyle choices impact their health.

5. Enhanced Healing: By addressing all aspects of a person's health, holistic health can enhance the body's natural healing processes. In Face Reflexology, this may result in faster recovery from illness, reduced pain, and improved overall well-being.

6. Emotional and Mental Well-being: Holistic health recognizes the importance of emotional and mental health in overall well-being. In Face Reflexology, this may involve techniques to reduce stress, promote relaxation, and improve mood.

7. Long-term Benefits: Holistic health aims to promote long-term health and well-being, rather than just providing temporary relief from symptoms. In Face Reflexology, this may involve lifestyle changes that support overall health and vitality.

In summary, holistic health is essential in Face Reflexology as it offers a comprehensive approach to health and well-being, addressing the physical, mental, emotional, and spiritual aspects of a person's health. By promoting balance and harmony in all areas of life, holistic health can help individuals achieve optimal health and well-being.

Diet and Lifestyle Recommendations for Overall Well-being

A holistic approach to well-being includes not just physical health but also mental, emotional, and spiritual well-being.

Here are some diet and lifestyle recommendations that can promote overall well-being:

1. Balanced Diet: Eat a variety of whole foods, including fruits, vegetables, whole grains, lean proteins, and healthy fats. Avoid processed foods, sugary drinks, and excessive amounts of caffeine and alcohol.

2. Hydration: Drink plenty of water throughout the day to stay hydrated and support overall health.

3. Regular Exercise: Engage in regular physical activity, such as walking, jogging, swimming, or yoga, to improve cardiovascular health, strengthen muscles, and boost mood.

4. Stress Management: Practice stress-reducing techniques such as meditation, deep breathing, yoga, or tai chi to reduce stress and promote relaxation.

5. Adequate Sleep: Aim for 7-9 hours of quality sleep each night to support overall health and well-being.

6. Social Connections: Maintain strong social connections with friends, family, and community members to support emotional well-being.

7. Mindfulness Practices: Practice mindfulness techniques such as meditation or yoga to cultivate a sense of presence and awareness in your daily life.

8. Limit Screen Time: Reduce screen time from devices such as smartphones, computers, and televisions to promote better sleep and reduce eye strain.

9. Creative Expression: Engage in creative activities such as writing, painting, or playing music to promote self-expression and reduce stress.

10. Nature Exposure: Spend time in nature regularly, whether it's a walk in the park or gardening, to improve mood and reduce stress.

11. Regular Health Check-ups: Schedule regular check-ups with your healthcare provider to monitor your health and address any concerns early.

12. Positive Relationships: Cultivate positive, supportive relationships with others to promote emotional well-being and reduce feelings of loneliness.

By incorporating these diet and lifestyle recommendations into your daily routine, you can promote overall well-being and enhance your quality of life.

The mind-body connection is a fundamental concept in Face Reflexology, as it acknowledges the intimate relationship between our physical health and our mental, emotional, and spiritual well-being.

Here's how the mind-body connection is understood and applied in Face Reflexology:

1. Physical Manifestation of Emotional States: Face Reflexology recognizes that emotional stress and tension can manifest physically in the body, including the face. By stimulating reflex points on the face, practitioners can help release emotional blockages and promote relaxation.

2. Stress Reduction: Face Reflexology can help reduce stress by stimulating reflex points that correspond to areas of tension in the face. This can help promote a sense of calmness and relaxation, which can have a positive impact on overall well-being.

3. Emotional Release: Just as physical tension can be released through reflexology, emotional tension can also be released. By stimulating reflex points on the face, practitioners can help clients release stored emotions and promote emotional healing.

4. Promotion of Mindfulness: During a Face Reflexology session, clients are encouraged to be present and mindful of the sensations in their face. This promotes a state of relaxation and can help reduce stress and anxiety.

5. Integration of Mind, Body, and Spirit: Face Reflexology views the individual as a whole, with the mind, body, and spirit interconnected.

By promoting balance and harmony in these areas, Face Reflexology can help enhance overall well-being.

6. Self-awareness: Through regular Face Reflexology sessions, individuals can become more aware of their facial tension patterns and how they may be related to their emotional state. This increased self-awareness can lead to greater emotional and physical well-being.

Overall, the mind-body connection is a central concept in Face Reflexology, highlighting the importance of addressing both physical and emotional aspects of health to promote holistic well-being.

CHAPTER 10

Face Reflexology Techniques

Advanced courses and training in Face Reflexology are available for practitioners who want to deepen their knowledge and skills in this specialized area. These courses often cover advanced techniques, specialized protocols for specific conditions, and ways to integrate Face Reflexology into a holistic health practice.

Here are some examples of advanced courses and training programs in Face Reflexology:

1. Advanced Face Reflexology Techniques: These courses focus on advanced techniques for stimulating reflex points on the face to address specific health concerns and promote overall well-being.

2. Specialized Protocols: Some courses offer specialized protocols for addressing common issues such as sinus congestion, headaches, and stress-related tension.

3. Integration with Other Modalities: Courses may also cover how to integrate Face Reflexology with other holistic health modalities, such as aromatherapy, acupressure, or massage therapy, to enhance treatment outcomes.

4. Anatomy and Physiology: Advanced courses may include a deeper dive into the anatomy and physiology of the face, including how reflex points correspond to different organs and systems in the body.

5. Client Assessment and Treatment Planning: Courses may cover how to conduct a thorough assessment of clients' needs and develop personalized treatment plans based on their individual health goals.

6. Ethics and Professionalism: Advanced training often includes topics related to ethics, professionalism, and client communication, ensuring that practitioners uphold high standards of practice.

7. Continuing Education: Many organizations offer continuing education courses and workshops for practitioners who want to stay updated on the latest research and techniques in Face Reflexology.

8. Certification Programs: Some advanced courses may lead to certification in Face Reflexology, demonstrating proficiency in advanced techniques and knowledge in the field.

Overall, advanced courses and training in Face Reflexology can provide practitioners with the skills and knowledge they need to enhance their practice and offer more comprehensive care to their clients.

Professional organizations and support groups can provide valuable resources, networking opportunities, and continuing education for practitioners of Face Reflexology.

Here are some organizations and groups that focus on holistic health and reflexology:

1. International Council of Reflexologists (ICR): The ICR is a global organization that promotes the practice of reflexology and provides resources and support for reflexologists worldwide.

2. American Reflexology Certification Board (ARCB): The ARCB is a certification board for reflexologists in the United States. They offer certification exams and continuing education opportunities for reflexologists.

3. Association of Reflexologists (AoR): The AoR is a UK-based organization that promotes the practice of reflexology and provides training, resources, and support for reflexologists in the UK and internationally.

4. Reflexology Association of Australia (RAoA): The RAoA is the peak body for reflexology in Australia. They provide training, resources, and support for reflexologists across Australia.

5. International Institute of Reflexology (IIR): The IIR is an organization that offers training and certification in reflexology. They also provide resources and support for reflexologists worldwide.

6. Reflexology Association of Canada (RAC): The RAC is a professional association for reflexologists in Canada. They offer training,

certification, and support for reflexologists across Canada.

7. National Association of Holistic Aromatherapy (NAHA): While not specific to reflexology, NAHA is a professional organization that promotes the safe use of aromatherapy and provides resources and support for holistic health practitioners.

These organizations and groups can be valuable resources for practitioners of Face Reflexology, providing access to education, certification, networking opportunities, and support from other professionals in the field.

CHAPTER 11

Summary of key points

In summary, Face Reflexology is a holistic therapy that focuses on stimulating reflex points on the face to promote healing and well-being. **Some key points about Face Reflexology include:**

1. Holistic Approach: Face Reflexology takes a holistic approach to health, recognizing the interconnectedness of the mind, body, and spirit.

2. Emotional Healing: By stimulating reflex points on the face, Face Reflexology can help release emotional blockages and promote emotional healing.

3. Stress Reduction: Face Reflexology can help reduce stress and promote relaxation by targeting reflex points that correspond to areas of tension in the face.

4. Beauty and Anti-Aging Benefits: Face Reflexology can promote beauty and anti-aging benefits by improving skin tone, reducing fine lines and wrinkles, and enhancing facial muscle tone.

5. Integration with Other Modalities: Face Reflexology can be integrated with other holistic health modalities, such as aromatherapy and massage therapy, to enhance treatment outcomes.

6. Advanced Training: Advanced courses and training programs are available for practitioners who want to deepen their knowledge and skills in Face Reflexology.

7. Professional Organizations: Professional organizations and support groups provide resources, networking opportunities, and continuing education for practitioners of Face Reflexology.

Overall, Face Reflexology offers a natural and effective way to promote healing and well-being, addressing both physical and emotional aspects of health.

Final Thoughts on Face Reflexology

Face Reflexology is a powerful and effective holistic therapy that can promote healing, relaxation, and overall well-being. By stimulating reflex points on the face, practitioners can help release tension, reduce stress, and promote emotional and physical healing. This gentle yet effective therapy offers a natural and non-invasive way to support health and vitality.

Encouragement for Continued Practice: For practitioners of Face Reflexology, your work is valuable and impactful. Each session you conduct has the potential to make a profound difference in the lives of your clients, promoting healing and enhancing their well-being. As you continue your practice, remember to stay curious, continue learning, and remain open to new techniques and approaches. Your dedication to your craft and your commitment to the health and well-being of others are truly commendable.

Keep up the great work, and may you continue to inspire healing and wellness in all that you do.

Glossary of Terms

Face Reflexology: A holistic therapy that involves stimulating reflex points on the face to promote healing and well-being.

Holistic Approach: An approach to health and wellness that considers the whole person, including physical, mental, emotional, and spiritual aspects.

Reflex Points: Points on the face that correspond to different organs, glands, and parts of the body.

Stress Reduction: The process of reducing stress levels in the body and mind, often through relaxation techniques and mind-body practices.

Emotional Healing: The process of addressing and healing emotional wounds and traumas, often through therapeutic interventions.

Beauty and Anti-Aging Benefits: The positive effects of Face Reflexology on skin tone, wrinkles, and overall appearance.

Advanced Training: Training programs that provide in-depth knowledge and skills in Face Reflexology beyond basic certification.

Professional Organizations: Organizations that provide support, resources, and networking opportunities for practitioners of Face Reflexology.

Continued Practice: The ongoing practice of Face Reflexology to maintain and improve skills and knowledge.

Client Assessment: The process of evaluating a client's health and wellness needs before a Face Reflexology session.

Lifestyle Recommendations: Recommendations for diet, exercise, sleep, and other lifestyle factors that can impact health and well-being.

Mind-Body Connection: The relationship between the mind and body, and how each can affect the other's health and well-being.

Integrative Approach: An approach to health that combines conventional and complementary therapies to promote healing and wellness.

Self-awareness: Awareness of one's own thoughts, feelings, and physical sensations, often cultivated through mindfulness practices.

Natural Healing: The body's ability to heal itself using its own resources and without the use of external interventions.

CONCLUSION

Congratulations on completing your journey through the world of Face Reflexology! As you close the pages of this compendium, you are equipped with the knowledge and techniques to embark on a lifelong practice that can transform your skin, body, and mind.

Reflecting on Your Journey: Throughout this book, you have learned about the ancient practice of Face Reflexology and its profound benefits for your overall health and well-being. You have explored the Face Reflexology map, learned how to locate and stimulate reflex points on your face, and discovered techniques to enhance relaxation, reduce stress, and improve your skin's health.

Embracing a Holistic Approach: At its core, Face Reflexology is not just about improving your skin's appearance or relieving tension. It is about embracing a holistic approach to health and well-being that recognizes the interconnectedness of your body, mind, and spirit. By practicing Face Reflexology, you are not only caring for your skin but also nurturing your entire being.

Continuing Your Practice: As you continue your journey with Face Reflexology, remember that consistency is key. Incorporate the techniques and principles you have learned into your daily life, and you will begin to see and feel the benefits. Whether you practice for a few minutes each day or dedicate longer sessions to your practice, the important thing is to listen to your body and respond to its needs.

Joining a Community: Consider joining a community or seeking out like-minded individuals who share your passion for Face Reflexology. By connecting with others, you can exchange tips, share experiences, and support each other on your journey to better health and well-being.

Final Thoughts: As you close this chapter on Face Reflexology, remember that the journey is ongoing. Your skin, body, and mind are constantly evolving, and Face Reflexology offers a lifelong path to self-discovery and self-care. Whether you are seeking to improve your skin's appearance, relieve stress, or simply enhance your overall well-being, Face Reflexology has something to offer you.

Thank you for allowing me to be your guide on this journey. May your practice of Face Reflexology bring you joy, peace, and radiant health for years to come.